Inspired Vegan Meals for Busy People

Tasty Dishes to Restart your Metabolism

Samantha Attanasio

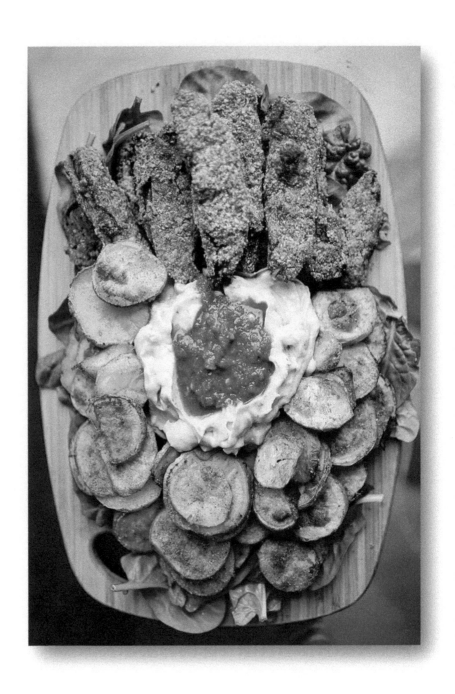

by reading this document, the reader agrees that under no circumstances is the author responsible for any losses, direct or indirect, which are incurred as a result of the use of information contained within this document, including, but not limited to, — errors, omissions, or inaccuracies.

Table of Contents

Vegetable

Florets and Pomegranate

Preparation time: 5 minutes

Cooking time: 7 minutes

Servings: 4

Ingredients:
- One broccoli head, florets separated
- Salt and black pepper to taste
- One pomegranate, seeds separated
- A drizzle of olive oil

Directions:

In a prepared bowl, mix the broccoli with the salt, pepper, and oil; toss.

Put the florets in your air fryer and cook at 400 degrees F for 7 minutes.

Divide between plates, sprinkle the pomegranate seeds all over and serve.

Nutrition:

Calories 141

Fat 3

Fiber 4

Carbs 11

Protein 4

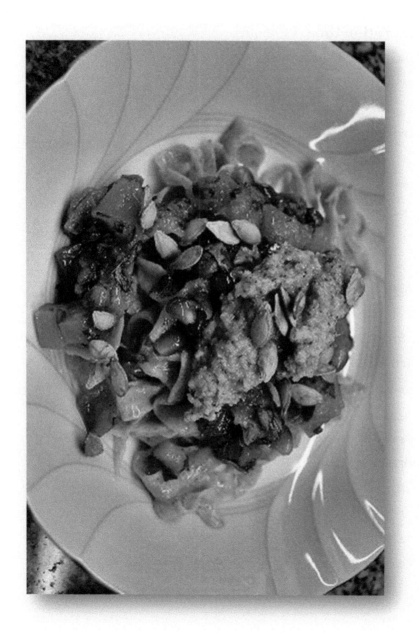

Lime Broccoli

Preparation time: 5 minutes

Cooking time: 6 minutes

Servings: 4

Ingredients:

- One broccoli head, florets separated
- One tbsp. lime juice
- Salt and black pepper to taste
- Two tbsp. vegan butter, melted

Directions:

In a prepared bowl, mix well all of the Ingredients.

Put the broccoli mixture in your air fryer and cook at 400 degrees F for 6 minutes.

Serve hot.

Nutrition:

Calories 151

Fat 4g

Fiber 7g

Carbs 12g

Protein 6g

Green Cayenne Cabbage

Preparation time: 5 minutes

Cooking time: 12 minutes

Servings: 4

Ingredients:

- One green cabbage head, shredded
- One tbsp. olive oil
- One tsp. cayenne pepper
- A pinch of salt and black pepper
- Two tsp. sweet paprika

Directions:

Mix all of the Ingredients in a pan that fits your fryer.

Place the pan in the fryer and cook at 320 degrees F for 12 minutes.

Divide between plates and serve right away.

Nutrition:

Calories 124

Fat 6g

Fiber 6g

Carbs 16g

Protein 7g

Tomato and Balsamic Greens

Preparation time: 5 minutes

Cooking time: 12 minutes

Servings: 4

Ingredients:

- One bunch mustard greens, trimmed
- Two tbsp. olive oil
- ½ cup veggies stock
- Two tbsp. tomato puree
- Three garlic cloves, minced
- Salt and black pepper to taste
- One tbsp. balsamic vinegar

Directions:

Combine all Ingredients in a pan that fits your air fryer and toss well. Place the pan in the fryer and cook at 260 degrees F for 12 minutes. Divide everything between plates, serve, and enjoy!

Nutrition:

Calories 151

Fat 2g

Fiber 4g

Carbs 14g

Protein 4g

Lime Endives

Preparation time: 5 minutes
Cooking time: 10 minutes
Servings: 4

Ingredients:

- Four endives, trimmed and halved
- Salt and black pepper to taste
- One tbsp. lime juice
- One tbsp. olive oil

Directions:

Put the endives in your air fryer, and add the salt, pepper, lemon juice, and vegan butter.

Cook at the temperature of 360 degrees F for 10 minutes.

Divide between plates and serve.

Nutrition:

Calories 100

Fat 3g

Fiber 4g

Carbs 8g

Protein 4g

Oregano Artichokes

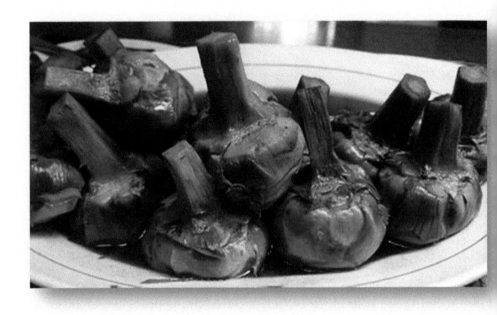

Preparation time: 10 minutes

Cooking time: 7 minutes

Servings: 4

Ingredients:

- Four big artichokes, trimmed
- Salt and black pepper to the taste
- Two tbsp. lemon juice
- ¼ cup extra virgin olive oil
- Two tsp. balsamic vinegar
- One tsp. oregano, dried
- 2 garlic cloves, minced

Directions:

Season the artichokes with salt and pepper, fry them with half the oil and half the lemon juice, place them in the air fryer and cook for seven minutes at 360 degrees F.

Meanwhile, in a bowl, mix the rest of the lemon juice with vinegar, the remaining oil, salt, pepper, garlic and oregano and stir very well.

Arrange artichokes on a platter, drizzle the balsamic vinaigrette over them and serve.

Enjoy!

Nutrition:

Calories 200

Fat 3g

Fiber 6g

Carbs 12g

Protein 4g

Green Veggies Mix

Preparation time: 10 minutes

Cooking time: 15 minutes

Servings: 4

Ingredients:

- 1-pint cherry tomatoes
- 1 pound green beans
- Two tbsp. olive oil
- Salt and black pepper to the taste

Directions:

In a bowl, mix cherry tomatoes with green beans, olive oil, salt and pepper, toss, transfer to your air fryer and cook at 400 degrees F for 15 minutes.

Divide among plates and serve right away.

Enjoy!

Nutrition:

Calories 162

Fat 6g

Fiber 5g

Carbs 8g

Protein 9g

Flavored Green Beans

Preparation time: 10 minutes
Cooking time: 15 minutes
Servings: 4

Ingredients:

- 1 pound red potatoes cut into wedges
- 1 pound green beans
- Two garlic cloves, minced
- Two tbsp. olive oil
- Salt and black pepper to the taste
- ½ tsp. oregano, dried

Directions:

In a pan that fits in air fryer, combine potatoes with green beans, garlic, oil, salt, pepper and oregano, toss, introduce in your air fryer and cook at 380 degrees F for 15 minutes.
Divide among plates and serve.
Enjoy!

Nutrition:
Calories 211
Fat 6g
Fiber 7g
Carbs 8g
Protein 5g

Beet Salad and Parsley Dressing

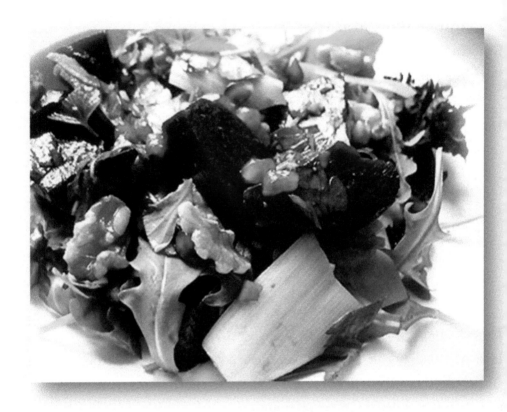

Preparation time: 10 minutes

Cooking time: 14 minutes

Servings: 4

Ingredients:

- Four beets
- 2 tbsp. balsamic vinegar
- A bunch of parsley

- Salt and black pepper
- 1 tbsp. extra virgin olive oil
- One garlic clove
- 2 tbsp. capers
-

Directions:

Insert beets in the air fryer and cook them at 360°F for 14 minutes.

Combine parsley with garlic, pepper, salt, olive oil and capers in a bowl and mix thoroughly

Move beets to a cutting board peel them after cooling and slice. Transfer them to a salad bowl.

Sprinkle the parsley dressing all over after putting in vinegar

Serve.

Nutrition:

Energy (calories): 27 kcal

Protein: 0.37 g

Fat: 1.58 g

Carbohydrates: 2.94 g

Beets and Arugula Salad

Preparation time: 5 minutes

Cooking time: 15 minutes

Servings: 4

Ingredients:

- One and ½ pounds beets
- A sprinkle of olive oil
- 2 tbsp. orange zest
- 2 tbsp. cider vinegar
- ½ cup of orange juice
- 2 tbsp. brown sugar
- Two scallions
- 2 tbsp. mustard
- 2 cups arugula

Directions:

Chafe beets with the orange juice and oil put in an air fryer and cook at 350° F for 10 minutes.

Move beet quarters to a bowl, put in arugula, orange Zest and scallions. Toss.

Blend sugar with mustard and vinegar in another bowl, beat well, and add to salad. Toss.

Serve.

Nutrition:

Energy (calories): 95 kcal

Protein: 2.78 g

Fat: 0.58 g

Carbohydrates: 20.76 g

Broccoli Salad

Preparation time: 5 minutes

Cooking time: 12 minutes

Servings: 4

Ingredients:

- One broccoli head, florets separated
- 1 tbsp. peanut oil
- Six garlic cloves
- 1 tbsp. Chinese rice wine vinegar
- Salt and black pepper

Directions:

Combine broccoli with salt, pepper and half of the oil in a bowl. Toss, put in an air fryer and cook at 350° F for 8 minutes while shaking fryer halfway.

Get broccoli to a salad bowl, put the garlic, the rest of the peanut oil, and rice vinegar. Toss thoroughly.

Serve.

Nutrition:

Energy (calories): 42 kcal

Fat: 3.43 g

Carbohydrates: 2.64 g

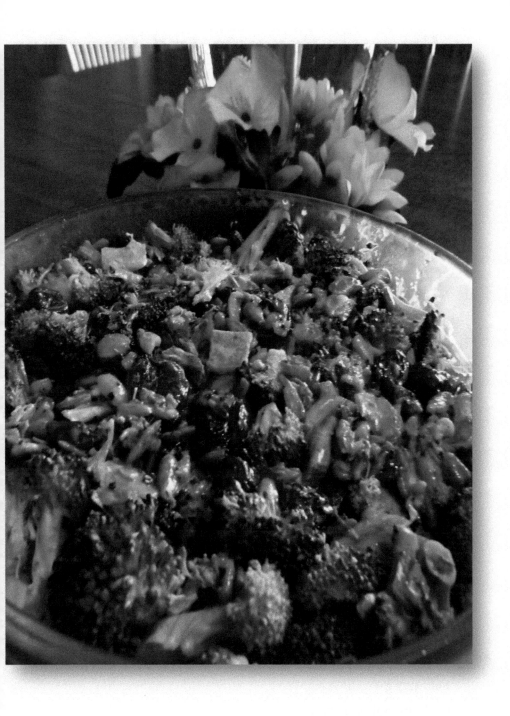

Brussels Sprouts And Tomatoes Mix

Preparation time: 5 minutes
Cooking time: 10 minutes
Servings: 4

Ingredients:

- 1 pound Brussels sprouts
- Salt and black pepper
- Six cherry tomatoes halved
- ¼ cup green onions,
- 1 tbsp. olive oil

Directions:

Spice Brussels sprouts with pepper and salt, get them in an Air Fryer. Cook at 350° F for 10 minutes.

Move them to a bowl; add cherry tomatoes, green onions, pepper, salt and olive oil. Toss properly

Serve.

Nutrition:

Energy (calories): 85 kcal
Protein: 4.04 g
Fat: 3.77 g
Carbohydrates: 11.52 g

Collard Green Mix

Preparation time: 5 minutes

Cooking time: 15 minutes

Servings: 4

Ingredients:

- One bunch collard greens
- 2 tbsp. olive oil
- 2 tbsp. tomato puree
- One yellow onion
- Three garlic cloves
- Salt and black pepper
- 1 tbsp. balsamic vinegar
- 1 tbsp. sugar

Directions:

Blend oil, vinegar, garlic, tomato puree and onion in a bowl and beat. Put in salt, pepper, collard greens and sugar. Toss, get it into the air fryer. Cook at 320° F for 10 minutes.

Share collard greens blend on plates

Serve.

Nutrition:

Energy (calories): 82 kcal

Protein: 0.46 g

Fat: 6.81 g

Carbohydrates: 5.24 g

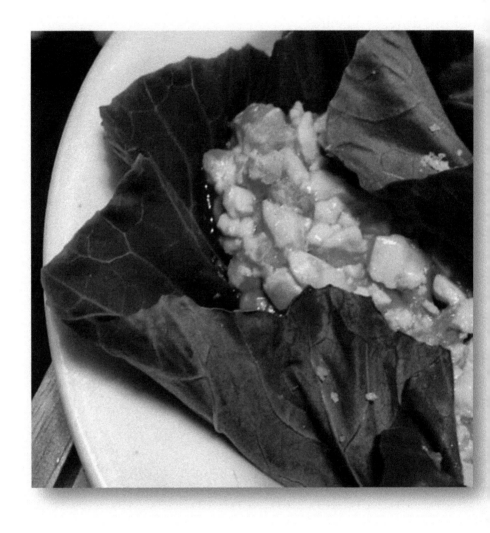

Herbed Eggplant and Zucchini Mix

Preparation time: 5 minutes
Cooking time: 13 minutes
Servings: 4

Ingredients:

- One eggplant, cubed
- Three zucchinis, cubed
- 2 tbsp. lemon juice
- Salt and black pepper
- 1 tbsp. dried thyme
- 1 tbsp. dried oregano
- 3 tbsp. olive oil

Directions:

Get a bowl, put in zucchinis, lemon juice, thyme pepper, salt, olive oil and oregano. Toss, put into the air fryer and cook at 360°F for 8 minutes.

Share in plates

Serve immediately.

Nutrition:

Energy (calories): 133 kcal

Protein: 1.79 g

Fat: 10.47 g

Carbohydrates: 10.1 g

Okra and Corn Salad

Preparation time: 5 minutes

Cooking time: 17 minutes

Servings: 6

Ingredients:

- 1-pound okra
- Six scallion s
- Three green bell peppers,
- Salt and black pepper
- 2 tbsp. olive oil
- 1 tbsp. sugar
- 28 oz. canned tomatoes
- 1 cup of corn

Directions:

Heat oil over medium heat in the pan, put bell peppers and scallion, turn and cook for 5 minutes.

Get in okra, pepper, salt, tomatoes, sugar and corn, stir, then put into the air fryer—Cook at 360° F for 7 minutes.

Share okra blend on plates.

Serve.

Nutrition:

Energy (calories): 209 kcal

Protein: 5.95 g

Fat: 6.38 g

Carbohydrates: 36.07 g

Crispy Potatoes and Parsley

Preparation time: 5 minutes
Cooking time: 15 minutes
Servings: 4

Ingredients:

- 1-pound gold potatoes, cut into wedges
- Salt and black pepper
- 2 tbsp. olive
- Juice from ½ lemon
- ¼ cup parsley leaves

Directions:

Pat potatoes with pepper, salt, lemon juice and olive oil, put into the air fryer, then cook at 350° F for 10 minutes.
Share in plates, spray parsley on top.
Serve.

Nutrition:

Energy (calories): 100 kcal
Protein: 2.63 g
Fat: 0.63 g
Carbohydrates: 21.84 g

Swiss Cha r d Salad

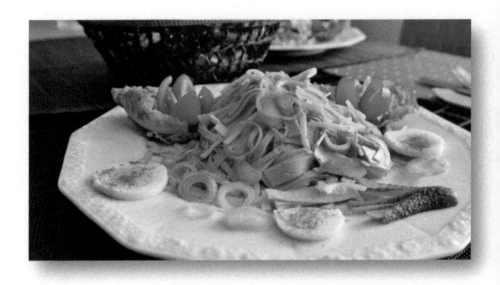

Preparation time: 5 minutes

Cooking time: 18 minutes

Servings: 4

Ingredients:

- One bunch Swiss chard
- 2 tbsp. olive oil
- One small yellow onion
- A pinch of red pepper flakes
- ¼ cup pine nuts
- ¼ cup raisins
- 1 tbsp. balsamic vinegar
- Salt and black pepper

Directions:

Heat pan and put olive oil over medium heat, put onions and chard, stir. Cook for 5 minutes.

Put pepper flakes, salt, pepper, raisins, vinegar and pine nuts, stir, bring into air fryer—Cook at 350° F for 8 minutes.

Share in plates

Serve.

Nutrition:

Energy (calories): 136 kcal

Protein: 1.76 g

Fat: 12.6 g

Carbohydrates: 5.62 g

Garlic Tomatoes

Preparation time: 5 minutes

Cooking time: 20 minutes

Servings: 4

Ingredients:

- Four garlic cloves
- 1 pound mixed cherry tomatoes
- Three thyme springs
- Salt and black pepper
- ¼ cup olive oil

Directions:

Mix in tomatoes with salt, garlic, black pepper, thyme and olive oil in a bowl. Toss to coat, bring into the air fryer. Cook at 360°F for 15 minutes.

Share tomatoes blend on plates

Serve.

Nutrition:

Energy (calories): 200 kcal

Protein: 1.56 g

Fat: 13.78 g

Carbohydrates: 20.26 g

Broccoli Hash

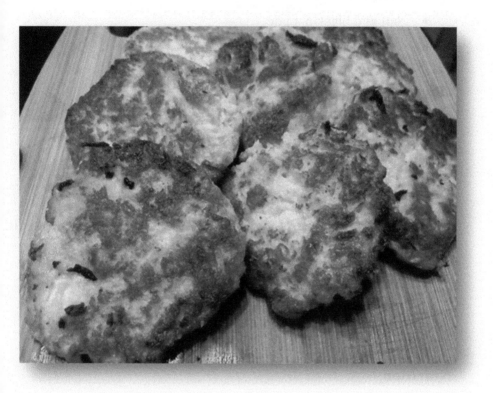

Preparation time: 10 minutes

Cooking time: 28 minutes

Servings: 2

Ingredients:

- 10 oz. mushrooms
- One broccoli head
- One garlic clov e
- 1 tbsp. balsamic vinegar

- One yellow onion
- 1 tbsp. olive oil
- Salt and black pepper
- 1 tbsp. dried basil
- One avocado
- A pinch of red pepper flakes

Directions:

Mix in mushrooms with onion, garlic, broccoli and avocado in a bowl.

Mix in oil, salt, pepper, vinegar and basil and beat properly.

Get this over veggies. Toss to coat, leave for 30 minutes. Put into air fryer's basket and then cook at 350° F for 8 minutes,

Share in plates.

Serve with pepper flakes over.

Nutrition:

Energy (calories): 280 kcal

Protein: 7.35 g

Fat: 22.1 g

Carbohydrates: 19.45 g

Eggplant and Garlic Sauce

Preparation time: 5 minutes
Cooking time: 15 minutes
Servings: 4

Ingredients:

- 2 tbsp. olive oil
- Two garlic cloves
- Three eggplants
- One red chilli pepper
- One green onion stalk
- 1 tbsp. ginger
- 1 tbsp. soy sauce
- 1 tbsp. balsamic vinegar

Directions:

Add eggplant slices to heated oil in the pan over medium heat and cook for 2 minutes.

Put in garlic, chilli pepper, green onions, soy sauce, ginger and Vinegar. Get into an air fryer and cook at 320° F for 7 minutes.

Share in plates.

Serve.

Nutrition:

Energy (calories): 186 kcal

Protein: 4.71 g

Fat: 8.27 g

Carbohydrates: 27.84 g

Stuffed Baby Peppers

Preparation time: 5 minutes
Cooking time: 11 minutes
Servings: 4

Ingredients:
- 12 baby bell peppers
- ¼ tbsp. red pepper flakes
- 6 tbsp. jarred basil pesto
- Salt and black pepper
- 1 tbsp. lemon juice
- 1 tbsp. olive oil
- Handful of parsley

Directions:

Mix in the pesto, salt, lemon juice, pepper flakes, black pepper, parsley and oil, beat properly and infuse bell pepper halves with the mix.
Put into the air fryer and then cook at 320° F for 6 minutes,
Assemble peppers on plates.
Serve.

Nutrition:

Energy (calories): 188 kcal
Protein: 25.86 g
Fat: 4.3 g
Carbohydrates: 14.52 g

Delicious Portobello Mushroom

Preparation time: 5 minutes

Cooking time: 17 minutes

Servings: 4

Ingredients:

- Ten basil leaves
- 1 cup baby spinach
- Three garlic cloves
- 1 cup almonds
- 1 tbsp. parsley
- ¼ cup olive oil
- Eight cherry tomatoes
- Salt and black pepper
- 4 Portobello mushrooms

Directions:

Blend basil with garlic, spinach, parsley, almonds, fat, black pepper, salt and mushroom. Mix thoroughly.

Infuse each mushroom with the blend, put them in an air fryer and cook at 350°F for 12 minutes .

Share mushrooms on plates.

Serve.

Nutrition:

Energy (calories): 135 kcal

Protein: 1.21 g

Fat: 13.8 g

Carbohydrates: 2.88 g

Cherry Tomatoes Skewers

Preparation time: 10 minutes

Cooking time: 26 minutes

Servings: 4

Ingredients:

- 3 tbsp. balsamic vinegar
- 24 cherry tomatoes
- 2 tbsp. olive oil
- Three garlic cloves
- 1 tbsp. thyme
- Salt and black pepper
- For dressing
- 2 tbsp. balsamic vinegar
- Salt and black pepper
- 4 tbsp. olive oil

Directions:

Mix in 2 tbsp. vinegar with three tbsp. oil, three garlic cloves, black pepper, thyme, salt in a bowl and beat properly.

Put tomatoes. Toss to coat and allow for 30 minutes.

Assemble six tomatoes on one skewer. Do the same with the remaining tomatoes.

Put into an air fryer and cook at 360°F for 6 minutes.

Mix in 2 tbsp. vinegar with salt, four tbsp. oil and pepper. Beat properly.

Assemble tomato skewers on plates.

Serve with dressing sprinkled over.

Nutrition:

Energy (calories): 210 kcal

Protein: 0.61 g

Fat: 20.34 g

Carbohydrates: 6.53 g

Green Beans and Tomatoes

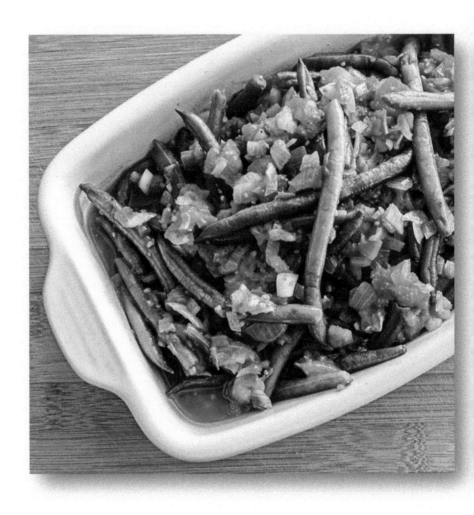

Preparation time: 5 minutes

Cooking time: 20 minutes

Servings: 4

Ingredients:

- 1-pint cherry tomatoes
- 1 lb. green beans
- 2 tbsp. Olive oil
- Salt and black pepper

Directions:

Mix in green beans with cherry potatoes, olive oil, pepper and salt.
Toss, put into the air fryer and cook at 400° F for 15 minutes.
Share in plates.
Serve immediately

Nutrition:

Energy (calories): 91 kcal
Protein: 1.46 g
Fat: 7.31 g
Carbohydrates: 6.34 g

Pumpkin Oatmeal

Preparation time: 5 minutes

Cooking time: 20 minutes

Servings: 4

Ingredients:

- Water (1.5 cups)
- Pumpkin puree (.5 cup)
- Stevia (3 tbsp.)
- Pumpkin pie spice (1 tsp.)
- Steel-cut oats (.5 cup)

Directions:

Set the Air Fryer at 360° Fahrenheit to preheat.

Toss in and mix the fixings into the pan of the Air Fryer.

Set the timer for 20 minutes.

When the time has elapsed, portion the oatmeal into bowls and serve.

Nutrition:

Calories 211

Protein 3 grams

Carbohydrates 1 gram

Fat 4 grams

Yellow Squash - Carrots & Zucchini

Preparation time: 5 minutes
Cooking time: 30 minutes
Servings: 4

Ingredients:

- Carrots (.5 lb.)
- Olive oil (6 tsp. - divided)
- Lime (1 sliced into wedges)
- Zucchini (1 lb. sliced into .75-inch semi-circles)
- Yellow squash (1 lb.)
- Tarragon leaves (1 tbsp.)
- White pepper (.5 tsp.)
- Sea salt (1 tsp.)

Directions:

Set the Air Fryer at 400° Fahrenheit.

Trim the stem and roots from the squash and zucchini.

Dice and add the carrots into a bowl with two teaspoons of oil.

Toss the carrots into the fryer basket. Prepare for 5 minutes.

Mix in the zucchini, oil, salt, and pepper in the bowl.

When the carrots are done, fold in the mixture. Cook 30 minutes.

Stir the mixture occasionally. Chop the tarragon and garnish using and lime wedges.

Nutrition:

Protein: 7.4 grams

Carbohydrates: 8.6 grams

Fat: 9.4 grams

Calories: 256

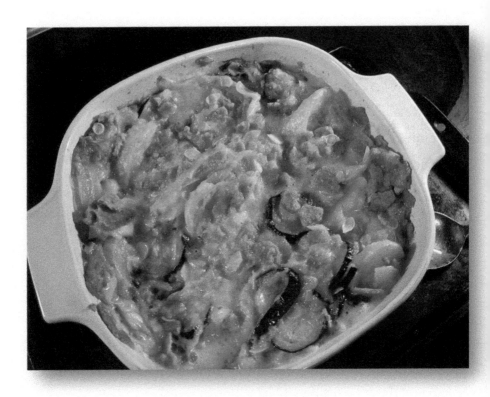

Carrot Mix

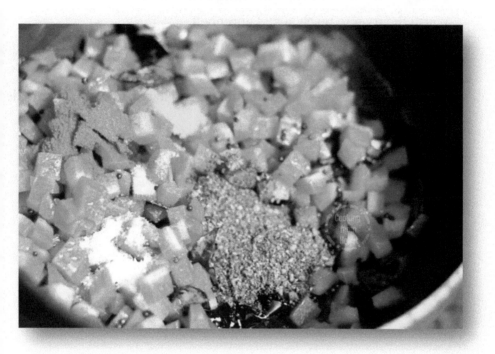

Preparation time: 5 minutes

Cooking time: 30 minutes

Servings: 4

Ingredients:

- Coconut milk (2 cups)
- Steel-cut oats (.5 cup)
- Shredded carrots (1 cup)
- Agave nectar (.5 tsp.)
- Ground cardamom (1 tsp.)
- Saffron (1 pinch)

48

Directions:

Lightly spritz the Air Fryer pan using a cooking oil spray.

Warm the fryer to reach 365° Fahrenheit.

When it's hot, whisk and add the fixings (omit the saffron).

Set the timer for 15 minutes.

After the timer buzzes, portion into the serving dishes with a sprinkle of saffron.

Nutrition:

Protein: 3 grams

Carbohydrates: 4 grams

Fat: 7 grams

Calories: 202

Vegan Fruits

Apple Pie Oatmeal Cookies

Preparation time: 10 minutes

Cooking time: 30 minutes

Servings: 4

Ingredients:

- 2 tsp. chia seeds or ground flax seeds
- 4 tbsp. of warm water
- 2 cup of regular or quick oats (use certified gluten-free if necessary)
- ¼ cup raisins
- 1 ½ tsp. pumpkin pie spice see Notes
- ½ tsp. baking soda
- ½ tsp. salt optional
- 1 large apple cored and chopped
- 2 ounces pitted and chopped dates (about four medjool dates or ¼ cup packed chopped dates)
- 1/8 cup water
- 1 tsp. apple cider vinegar

Directions:

Preheat the oven to 375.

In a prepared small bowl, combine the chia seeds (or ground flaxseed) with the warm water and set aside until thickened.

In a dry blender or food processor, grind one cup of the oats. Pour it into a mixing bowl and add the unground oats, pumpkin pie spice, baking soda, and salt. Stir in the raisins.

Place the apple, dates, 1/8 cup water, and apple cider vinegar in the blender. Blend until the consistency of apple sauce is about it. Pour it together with the chia "egg" or egg replacer flax egg into the oat mixture and whisk to blend.

Fall through the rounded tbsp. Onto a baking sheet lined with parchment paper or a silicon mat. With a fork, flatten each cookie slightly. For about 12 minutes, bake. Until serving, cool on a wire rack.

Nutrition:

Energy (calories): 225 kcal

Protein: 5.86 g

Fat: 2.87 g

Carbohydrates: 46.23 g

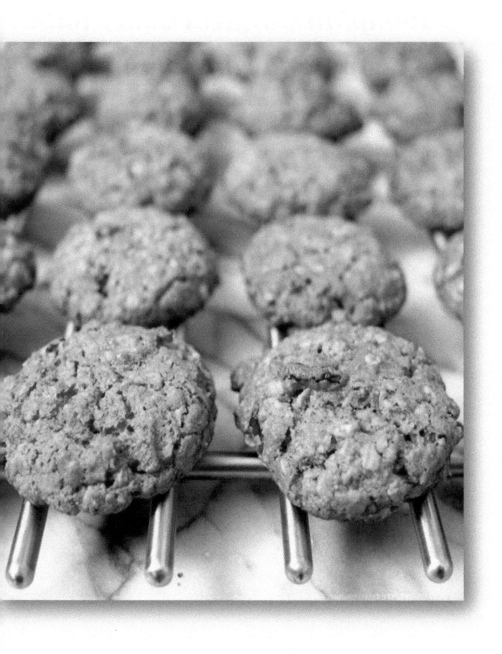

Pumpkin Oatmeal Cakes with Apple-Pecan Compote

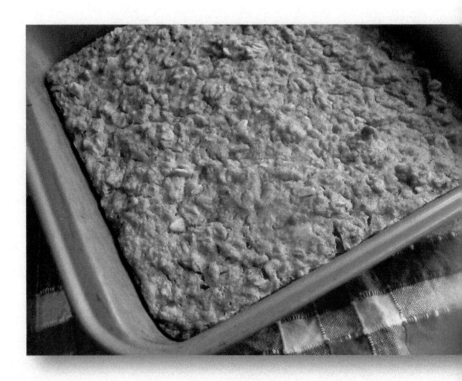

Preparation time: 10 minutes

Cooking time: 30 minutes

Servings: 4

Ingredients:

- 2 cups water
- ½ cup chopped dates about 3 ounces

- ¾ cups canned pumpkin
- ¾ tsp. cinnamon
- ¼ tsp. allspice
- ¼ tsp. powdered ginger
- ½ tsp. salt
- 1 tbsp. ground flaxseed
- 1 ½ cups steel-cut oats
- 1 ¼ cup plain coconut milk (the drinking kind, not canned) or other non-dairy milk
- non-stick spray

Directions:

In a blender, put the water and dates and blend until the dates are finely chopped. Add the pumpkin, herbs, flaxseed and salt and blend until well mixed.

Heat a large saucepan and toast the oats, stirring periodically, for 1-2 minutes, until fragrant. The pumpkin mixture is carefully applied, standing back in case it spatters, and then the coconut milk. Stir well, reduce the heat to medium, and cook for about 30 minutes or until thick and chewy, stirring frequently.

Line an 11×7-inch baking dish with parchment paper or spray with non-stick spray. Spread the oats in the container, smoothing the top. Cool on the counter for one hour and then refrigerate until thoroughly chilled, at least an hour. Put onto a cutting board and cut into 16 triangles or rectangles.

Spray into a large non-stick frying pan with a light coating of vegan cooking spray and heat over medium-high heat. Add half of the oatmeal cakes and cook on each side until lightly browned, 2-3 minutes per side. Remove to a warm oven and repeat with the remaining patties. Keep warm until ready to serve.

Place two cakes on each dessert plate. Top with warm Apple-Pecan Compote, below.

Nutrition:

Energy (calories): 453 kcal

Protein: 15.37 g

Fat: 32.39 g

Carbohydrates: 45.8 g

Peach Oatmeal Bars

Preparation time: 10 minutes
Cooking time: 20 minutes
Servings: 4

Ingredients:

- 2 cups old fashioned or rolled oats
- ¼ cup chopped dates
- 2 tbsp. chopped almonds
- 1 tbsp. chia seed or ground flax seeds
- 1 tsp. baking powder
- 1 tsp. cinnamon
- 1/8 tsp. pure stevia extract powder optional
- ¾ cup plus two tbsp. non-dairy milk I used vanilla soymilk
- 2 peaches about one ¼ cups, peeled and diced
- 1 tsp. vanilla
- ¼ tsp. almond extract

Directions:

Preheat oven to 350F. Line an 8×8- or 9×9-inch baking pan with parchment paper (this makes sure they don't stick and makes clean-up a breeze).

Combine dry Ingredients (oats through stevia) in a large bowl. In a medium bowl, combine the remaining Ingredients. Stir the wet Ingredients into the dry, making sure that they are thoroughly combined. Spread into prepared pan. Bake for about 25 minutes. If you'd like a crunchier top, put the pan under the broiler for a minute or two, observing to make sure they don't burn.

Remove from oven and allow to cool for at least 15 minutes. Remove from pan by lifting parchment paper. Cut into nine squares and enjoy.

Nutrition:

Energy (calories): 295 kcal

Protein: 10.76 g

Fat: 5.11 g

Carbohydrates: 72.51 g

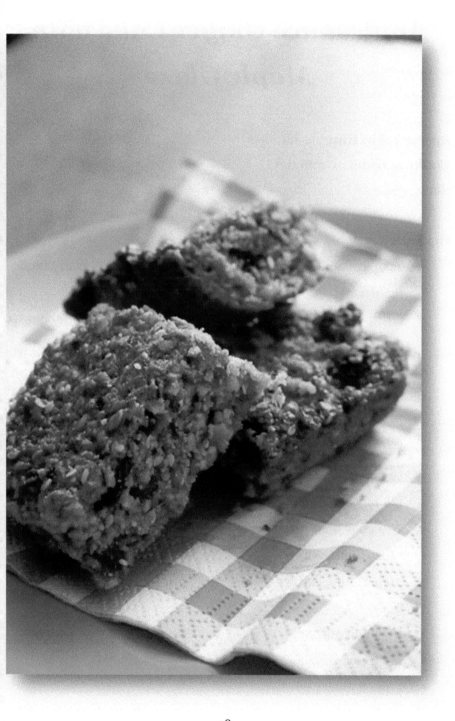

Applesauce Ginger Cake with Maple Glaze

Preparation time: 10 minutes

Cooking time: 40 minutes

Servings: 4

Ingredients:

- 2 cups of white whole wheat flour or whole wheat pastry flour
- 1 cup sugar
- 2 tbsp. crystallized (candied) ginger, chopped small (about ¾ ounce)
- 1 tbsp. cornstarch
- 2 tsp. baking soda
- 1 ½ tsp. ginger powder
- ½ tsp. salt
- ½ tsp. cinnamon
- 1/8 tsp. cloves
- 2 ¼ cups unsweetened applesauce
- 1 tbsp. lemon juice
- 1 tsp. vanilla extract
- Glaze
- ¼ cup maple syrup
- 1 tsp. cornstarch
- 1 pinch ginger powder

- Additional candied ginger for serving optional

Directions:

Preheat oven at temperature of 350 degrees F. Lightly oil a bundt pan or 9×9-inch baking pan.

Mix all the dry Ingredients; then add the applesauce, lemon juice, and vanilla extract. Stir until combined but don't over-stir. Pour into a pan and then bake for 45-60 minutes. By inserting a toothpick into the center test it; it's done when the toothpick comes out perfectly clean . Remove from air fryer oven and let it cool for 10 minutes. Invert onto a cake dish.

Prepare the glaze: Combine the maple syrup, one tsp. cornstarch, and a generous pinch of powdered ginger in a small saucepan and mix well. Bring and let it boil over medium-high heat, continuously stirring. 1 minute to simmer. Remove from heat and allow to thicken and cool. (In order to speed up the cooling, you should put the pan in a bowl of cold water.) When the glaze has thickened but is still pourable, drizzle it over the cake. Serve immediately, garnished with strips, if desired, of candied ginger.

Nutrition:

Energy (calories): 451 kcal

Protein: 6.8 g

Fat: 0.8 g

Carbohydrates: 105.08 g

Vegan Dessert

Rose Meringue Kisses

The first time I learned of infusing rose into food, I couldn't wait to try my hands on it. Here is a simple, pink specialty that you'll love. Your little girls will enjoy making them with you.

Preparation time: 7 minutes

Cooking time: 40 minutes

Servings: 4

Ingredients:

- ¼ cup aquafaba
- 4 tbsp. caster sugar
- ½ tsp. rose water
- Pink food colouring

Directions:

Pour the aquafaba into a bowl and whisk with an electric mixer until a soft peak forms.

Gradually, add the sugar while whisking until well-combined. Fold in the rose water and pink food colouring to achieve the intensity of pink color as desired.

Mix the combined mixture into a piping bag and squeeze out mounds on a cookie sheet that fits into the fryer basket.

Preheat the air fryer and bake the meringues at 200 F for 40 minutes or until the meringues are firm like a biscuit.

Remove to cool and serve.

Nutrition:

Calories 100

Total Fat 7g

Total Carbs 7g

Fiber 0g

Net Carbs 7g

Protein 2g

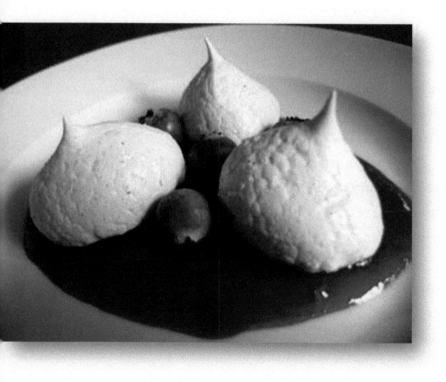

Three – Ingredient Shortbread Biscuits

Preparation time: 10 minutes

Cooking time: 12 minutes

Servings: 4

Ingredients:

- 1/3 cup melted vegan butter
- 3 tbsp. caster sugar
- ½ cup flour

Directions:

In a bowl, combine the Ingredients until well mixed.

Place the flour on a chopping board and knead until smooth and pleasant.

Cut into finger bites and decorate with fork holes.

Preheat the air fryer and put the bites in the fryer basket—Bake at 350 F for 12 minutes.

Terrific turnout!

Nutrition:

Calories 245

Total Fat 15g

Total Carbs 26g

Fiber 2g

Net Carbs 24g

Protein 2g

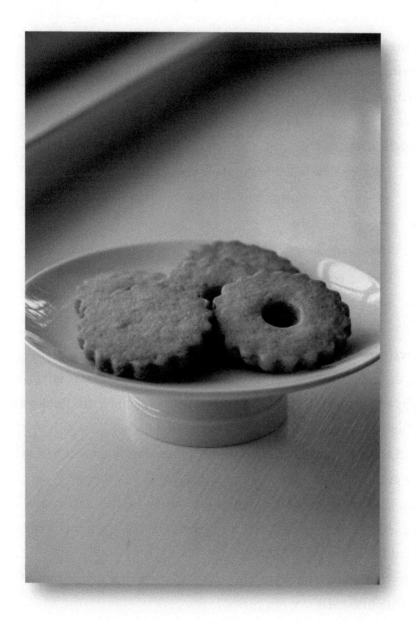

Molten Chocolate and Peanut Butter Fondants

Preparation time: 15 minutes
Cooking time: 7 minutes
Servings: 4

Ingredients:

- 1 cup unsweetened vegan dark chocolate
- 4 tbsp. vegan butter, diced divided
- 5 tbsp. aquafaba
- 1/8 cup flour
- ½ cup confectioner's sugar, divided
- 1 tsp. salt

Directions:

Pour the chocolate, half of the vegan butter in a bowl and microwave until completely melted. Stir at every 10-seconds interval. Remove the bowl and allow slight cooling.

Add in the aquafaba and whisk while adding the flour and half of the sugar gradually. Set aside.

In another bowl, melt the remaining butter in the microwave and whisk with the peanut butter and the remaining confectioner's sugar.

Preheat the air fryer.

Grease four small ramekins with cooking spray and divide half of the chocolate into each.

Pour the peanut butter into each ramekin's center and pour the remaining chocolate on top to cover the peanut butter.

Place two ramekins in the fryer basket and bake at 300 F for 7 minutes.

Remove and cook the remaining batter.

Cool for a minute, turn the fondants over onto plates and enjoy the delight.

Nutrition:

Calories 504

Total Fat 39g

Total Carbs 29g

Fiber 1g

Net Carbs 28g

Protein 10g

Raspberry Mug Cakes

Preparation time: 5 minutes

Cooking time: 5 minutes

Servings: 4

Ingredients:

- ¼ cup flour
- 1 tsp. baking powder
- 5 tbsp. sugar
- ½ cup chopped dairy-free white chocolate, melted
- 4 tbsp. almond milk
- 3 tsp. melted vegan butter
- 1 tsp. vanilla extract
- A pinch sal t
- ½ cup raspberries

Directions:

In a bowl, mix all the Ingredients except the raspberries until properly combined and pour into four mugs, leaving 1 – inch space on top for rising.

Divide the raspberries into the mugs and fold into the mixture.

Place 2 cups in the fryer basket and bake at 380 F for 5 minutes or until the cakes are set.

Remove and cook the remaining batter.

Allow cooling and serve.

Nutrition:

Calories 186

Total Fat 13g

Total Carbs 8g

Fiber 0g

Net Carbs 8g

Protein 9g

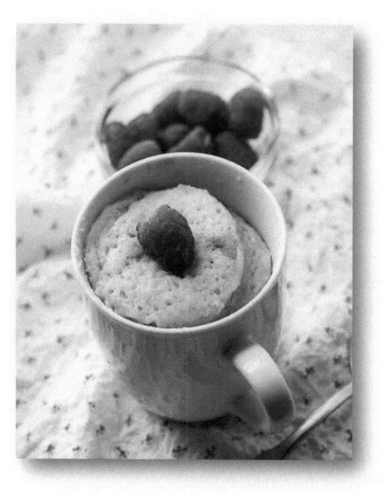

Yogurt Soufflé

Preparation time: 25 minutes

Cooking time: 14 minutes

Servings: 2

Ingredients:

- 1 tbsp. unbelted vegan butter
- ¼ cup of sugar
- 1 cup dairy-free yogurt
- A pinch salt
- ¼ tsp. vanilla extract
- 3 tbsp. flour
- ½ cup aquafaba
- 3 oz. dairy-free coconut heavy cream

Directions:

Coat two 6-oz ramekins with the vegan butter.

Pour in the sugar and swirl in the ramekins to coat the butter. Pour out the remaining sugar and reserve.

Melt the remaining vegan butter in a microwave and set aside.

In a bowl, whisk the butter, yogurt, salt, vanilla extract, flour, and half of the aquafaba. Set aside.

In another bowl, beat the remaining aquafaba with the coconut cream until foamy.

Fold the coconut cream mixture into the yogurt mix one-third portion at a time as you thoroughly combine.

Preheat the air fryer.

Share the mix into the ramekins with ½-inch space left on top.

Put the ramekins in the fryer basket and bake at 350 F for 14 minutes.

When ready, remove and serve.

Nutrition:

Calories 251

Total Fat 18g

Total Carbs 18g

Fiber 2g

Net Carbs 16g

Protein 4g

Fried Oreos

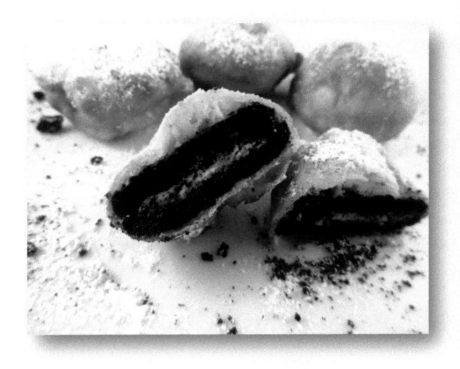

Preparation time: 50 minutes

Cooking time: 10 minutes

Servings: 4

Ingredients:

- 16 Oreo cookies
- 1 cup eggless pancake mix
- 2/3 cup almond milk
- 3 tbsp. flax egg
- 2 tsp. olive oil
- Confectioner's sugar for dusting

Directions:

Freeze the Oreo cookies for 45 minutes.

In a bowl, combine the remaining Ingredients until combined evenly.

Preheat the air fryer and grease the fryer basket with cooking spray.

Get the cookies from the fridge and coat deeply in the batter so that you cannot see through the batter.

Place the cookies in the fryer basket and fry at 350 F for 10 minutes or until a biscuit forms.

Transfer the cookies to a plate, relaxed for a few minutes, and dust with the sugar.

Serve.

Nutrition:

Calories 98

Total Fat 2g

Total Carbs 4g

Fiber 0g

Net Carbs 6g

Protein 16g

Plum Cobbler

Preparation time: 5 minutes

Cooking time: 12 minutes

Servings: 2

Ingredients:

- ¼ cup of sugar
- ¼ cup flour
- ½ cup cornmeal
- 1 tbsp. baking powder
- A pinch of salt
- 4 tbsp. melted vegan butter + extra for greasing
- 1 tsp. vanilla extract
- 4 tbsp. plant milk (non-dairy milk)
- 2 cups stewed plums
- 1 tsp. lemon juice

Directions:

In a bowl, mix the sugar, flour, cornmeal, baking powder, vegan butter, vanilla extract, and non-dairy milk until smoothly combined.

Grease a 3 x 3 baking dish with the remaining butter and pour in the plums with lemon juice. Stir to combine.

Spoon the flour mixture on top and use a spoon to level the mix.

Place the dish in the fryer basket and bake at 390 F for 12 minutes.

Remove after; allow cooling for a few minutes, and serve with vegan ice cream.

Nutrition:

Calories 180

Total Fat 14g

Total Carbs 10g

Fiber 2g

Net Carbs 8g

Protein 3g

Vegan Snacks

Crispy Brussels Sprouts

Preparation time: 5 minutes

Cooking time: 1 minute

Servings: 2

Ingredients:

- 2 cups Brussels sprouts, sliced
- 1 tbsp. olive oil
- 1 tbsp. balsamic vinegar
- Salt to taste

Directions:

Toss all the Ingredients in a bowl.

Cook in the air fryer at 400 degrees F for 10 minutes. Shake once or twice during the cooking process.

Check to see if crispy enough.

If not, cook for another 5 minutes.

Nutrition:

Calories 100

Total Fat 7.3g

Total Carbohydrate 8.1g

Dietary Fiber 3.3g

Protein 3g

Sweet Potato Tots

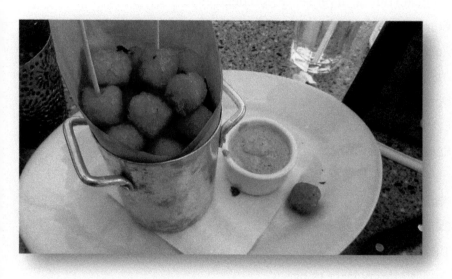

Preparation time: 10 minutes

Cooking time: 12 minutes

Servings: 10

Ingredients:

- 2 cups sweet potato puree
- ½ tsp. salt
- ½ tsp. cumin
- ½ tsp. coriander
- ½ cup breadcrumbs
- Cooking spray
- Vegan mayo

Directions:

Preheat your air fryer set to 390 degrees F.

Combine all Ingredients in a bowl.

Form into balls.

Arrange on the air fryer pan.

Spray with oil.

Cook for 6 minutes or until golden.

Serve with vegan mayo.

Nutrition:

Calories 77

Total Fat 0.8g

Total Carbohydrate 15.9g

Dietary Fiber 1.1g

Total Sugars 3.1g

Protein 1.8g

Popcorn Tofu

Preparation time: 15 minutes

Cooking time: 12 minutes

Servings: 4

Ingredients:

- ½ cup cornmeal
- ½ cup quinoa flour
- 1 tbsp. vegan bouillon
- 2 tbsp. Nutritional yeast
- 1 tsp. garlic powder
- 1 tsp. onion powder
- 1 tbsp. mustard
- Salt and pepper to taste
- ¾ cup almond milk
- 1 ½ cups breadcrumbs
- 14 oz. tofu, sliced into small pieces
- ½ cup vegan mayo
- 2 tbsp. hot sauce

Directions:

In the first bowl, mix the first eight Ingredients.

In the second bowl, pour the almond milk.

In the third bowl, add the breadcrumbs.

Dip each tofu slice into each of the bowls starting from the flour mixture, then the almond milk, and finally, the breadcrumbs.

Cook in the air fryer set the temperature at 350 degrees F for 12 minutes, shaking halfway through.

Mix the mayo and hot sauce and serve with tofu.

Nutrition:

Calories 261

Total Fat 5.5 g

Total Carbohydrate 37.5 g

Dietary Fiber 4.8 g

Protein 16 g

Black Bean Burger

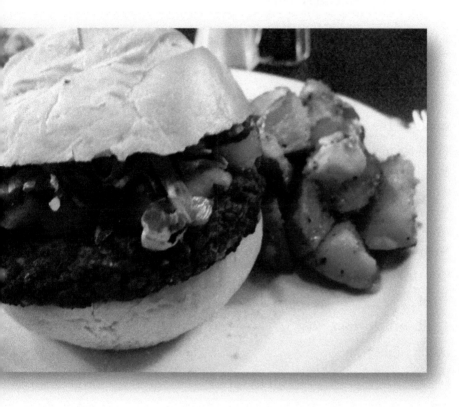

Preparation time: 10 minutes

Cooking time: 25 minutes

Servings: 6

Ingredients:

- One ¼ cup rolled oats
- 16 oz. black beans, rinsed and drained
- ¾ cup of salsa
- 1 tbsp. soy sauce

- One ¼ tsp. chilli powder
- ¼ tsp. chipotle chilli powde r
- ½ tsp. garlic powder

Directions:

Pulse the oats inside a food processor until powdery.

Apply all the remaining Ingredients and pulse until well combined.

Transfer to a bowl and refrigerate for 15 minutes.

Form into burger patties.

Cook in the air fryer at 375 degrees F for 15 minutes.

Nutrition:

Calories 158

Total Fat 2 g

Total Carbohydrate 30 g

Dietary Fiber 9 g

Protein 8 g

Vegan Bread and Pizza

Vegan Caprese Sandwiches

Usually, a classic Caprese salad is served with a crisp artisan bread so you can sop up the flavours. Now enjoy that delicious salad in sandwich form! Don't overlook the last drizzle of olive oil on the sandwich bread: it pulls all of those traditional flavours together.

Preparation time: 10 minutes
Cooking time: 10 minutes
Servings: 2

Ingredients:

- 2 tbsp. balsamic vinegar
- 4 slices gluten-free sandwich bread
- 2 ounces vegan mozzarella shreds
- Two medium Roma tomatoes, sliced
- Eight fresh basil leaves
- 2 tbsp. olive oil

Directions:

Preheat the air fryer and set the temperature at 350°F for 3 minutes. Prepare sandwiches by drizzling balsamic vinegar on bottom bread slices: layer mozzarella, tomatoes, and basil leaves on top. Add top bread slices.

Brush outside the top and bottom of each sandwich lightly with olive oil. Place one sandwich in an ungreased air fryer basket and cook for 3 minutes. Flip and cook an additional 2 minutes—transfer the sandwich to a large serving plate and repeat with the second sandwich.

Serve warm.

Nutrition:

Energy (calories): 440 kcal

Protein: 17.93 g

Fat: 22.6 g

Carbohydrates: 41.19 g

Mini Mushroom-Onion Eggplant Pizzas

Preparation time: 5 minutes
Cooking time: 16 minutes
Servings: 4

Ingredients:

- 2 tsp. + 2 tbsp. olive oil, divided
- 1/4 cup small-diced peeled yellow onion
- 1/2 cup small-diced white mushrooms
- 1/2 cup marinara sauce
- One small eggplant, sliced into 8 (1/2") circles
- 1 tsp. salt
- 1 cup vegan shredded mozzarella
- 1/4 cup chopped fresh basil

Directions:

In a prepared medium skillet over medium heat, heat 2 tsp. olive oil 30 seconds. Add onion and mushrooms and cook for 5 minutes until onions are translucent. Add marinara sauce and stir. Remove skillet from heat.

Preheat the air fryer at 375°F for 3 minutes.

Rub remaining olive oil over both sides of eggplant circles. Lay circles on a large plate and season top evenly with salt—top with marinara sauce mixture, followed by shredded mozzarella.

Place half of the eggplant pizzas in an ungreased air fryer basket. Cook 5 minutes.

Transfer cooked pizzas to a large plate. Repeat with remaining pizzas. Garnish with chopped basil and serve warm.

Nutrition:

Energy (calories): 111 kcal

Protein: 10.94 g

Fat: 3.15 g

Carbohydrates: 11.74 g

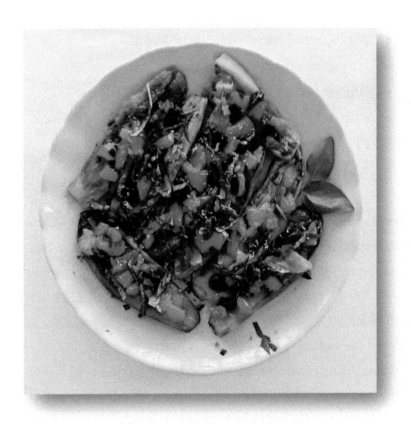

Cauliflower Personal Pizza Crusts

Preparation time: 10 minutes
Cooking time: 30 minutes
Servings: 2

Ingredients:

- 1 cup cauliflower rice
- 1 1/2 tbsp. Tapioca starch
- 1/2 cup vegan grated mozzarella
- One clove garlic, peeled and minced
- 1 tsp. Italian seasoning
- 1/8 tsp. salt

Directions:

Preheat and set the air fryer's temperature to 400°F for 3 minutes.

In a medium bowl, combine all Ingredients.

Divide mixture in half and spread into two pizza pans lightly greased with preferred cooking oil.

Place one pan in an air fryer basket and cook for 12 minutes. Once done, remove the pan from the basket and repeat with the second pan. Top crusts with your favourite toppings and cook an additional 3 minutes.

Nutrition:

Energy (calories): 86 kcal

Protein: 10.16 g

Fat: 0.16 g

Carbohydrates: 11.33 g

Pizza Bombs

Preparation time: 5 minutes
Cooking time: 12 minutes
Servings: 9 pizza bites

Ingredients:

- 1/3 cup gluten-free all-purpose flour
- 1/4 tsp. salt
- 1/4 tsp. baking powder
- 1/2 cup small-diced pepperoni
- 2 ounces Tofutti, room temperature
- 1/4 cup vegan shredded mozzarella cheese
- 1/2 tsp. Italian seasoning
- 2 tbsp. Almond Milk
- 1 tsp. olive oil
- 1/2 cup vegan marinara sauce, warmed

Directions:

Preheat the air fryer at 325°F for 5 minutes.

In a small bowl, combine flour, salt, and baking powder.

In a prepared medium bowl, combine the remaining Ingredients, except vegan marinara sauce, mixing until smooth. Add dry Ingredients to bowl and mix until well combined.

Form mixture into nine (1") balls and place on an ungreased pizza pan. It's okay if pizza balls are touching. Put the pan in air fryer basket and cook 12 minutes.

Transfer balls to a large plate. Serve warm with vegan marinara sauce on the side for dipping.

Nutrition:

Energy (calories): 112 kcal

Protein: 4.49 g

Fat: 3.94 g

Carbohydrates: 14.85 g

Vegan Main Dishes

Creamy Cauliflower and Broccoli

"One of the best Air Fryer salad you are ever going to taste! Cauliflower and broccoli mixed with cashew cheese. Creamy heaven!"

Preparation time: 5 minutes

Cooking time: 16 minutes

Servings: 6

Temperature: 390degreesF

Ingredients:

- 1-pound cauliflower florets
- One tbsp. lemon zest, grated
- Two and ½ tbsp. sesame oil
- ¾ tsp. sea salt flakes
- ½ cup cashew cheese
- 1-pound broccoli florets
- ½ tsp. cayenne pepper, smoked

Directions:

Preheat your Air Fryer and set the temperature at 390 degrees F

Prepare the cauliflower and broccoli using the steaming method

Drain it and add cayenne pepper, sesame oil, and salt flakes

Cook for 15 minutes

Check your vegetables halfway during cooking

Stir in the lemon zest and cashew cheese

Toss to coat well

Serve warm and enjoy!

Nutrition:

Calories: 133

Fat: 9.0g

Carbohoydrates: 7g

Protein: 5.9g

Roasted Chickpeas

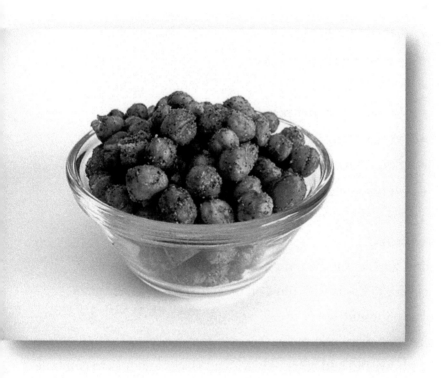

"The mango powder here really helps to flavour up the chickpeas here while the cinnamon and cumin bring them all so needed heat! Lovely."

Preparation time: 2 minutes
Cooking time: 10 minutes
Servings: 4
Temperature: 390degreesF

Ingredients:

- ¼ tsp. Mango powder, dried
- ½ tsp. Cinnamon powder
- ¼ tsp. cumin powder
- 3 cups chickpeas, boiled
- 1 tsp. Salt
- ¼ tsp. Coriander powder, dried
- ½ tsp. chilli powder
- 1 tsp. Olive oil
- ¼ tsp. rosemary

Directions:

Preheat and set the air fryer's temperature to 370 degrees F

Transfer chickpeas with olive oil in your Air Fryer basket

Cook for 8 minutes

Shake after every 2 minutes

Take a bowl and add chickpeas with all spices and toss to combine

Serve and enjoy!

Nutrition:

Calories: 214

Fat: 4.4g

Carbohoydrates: 34.27g

Protein: 10.98g

Rosemary Russet Potato Chips

"Rosemary flavoured russet potatoes, just one of the many ways of preparing your amazing potatoes!"

Preparation time: 10 minutes
Cooking time: 60 minutes
Servings: 4
Temperature: 330degreesF

Ingredients:

- Four russet potatoes
- ½ tsp. salt
- 2 tsp. rosemary, chopped
- 1 tbsp. olive oil

Directions:

Rinse potatoes and scrub to clean

Peel and cut them in a lengthwise manner similar to thin chips

Take a bowl and put them into it and soak water for 30 minutes

Take another bowl and toss the chips with olive oil

Transfer them to the cooking basket

Cook for 30 minutes at 330 degrees F

Toss with salt and rosemary while warm

Enjoy!

Nutrition:

Calories: 322

Fat: 3.69g

Carbohoydrates: 66g

Protein: 7.5g

Vegan Staples

Rainbow Veggies

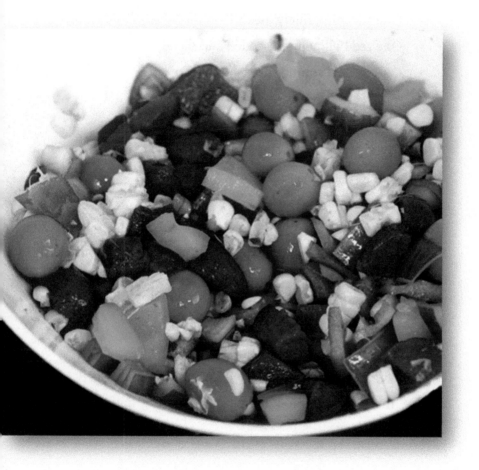

Rainbow Veggies made in the air fryer caramelize in a lovely way without overcooking. Toss them with your favourite vinaigrette, mixed with greens for a different salad.

Preparation time: 10 minutes

Cooking time: 20 minutes

Servings: 4

Ingredients:

- One zucchini, finely diced
- One red bell pepper, seeded and diced
- One yellow summer squash, finely diced
- ½ sweet white onion, finely diced
- 4 oz. fresh mushrooms, cleaned and halved
- 1 tbsp. extra-virgin olive oil
- Salt and pepper, to taste

Directions:

Preheat the air fryer according to the recommendations of the air fryer.

Place the red bell pepper, zucchini, mushrooms, squash and onion in a large bowl.

Add the olive oil, black pepper and salt, and toss to combine.

Place the vegetables in a single layer in the air fryer basket.

Air-fry, the vegetables for 20 minutes, stirring halfway through the Cooking time.

Nutrition:

Total Calories: 69 kcal.

Carbohydrates 7.7g

Protein 2.6g

Fat 3.8g

Sodium 48mg

Cholesterol 0mg

Tofu with Carrots and Broccoli

With an air-fryer, Chinese take-out is simple and nutritious. In an orange sauce, the crispy tofu is tossed with plenty of vegetables. It's easy to make and has less oil in it. {Vegan, Adaptable to Gluten-Free}

Preparation time: 10 minutes

Cooking time: 15 minutes

Servings: 2

Ingredients:

- For the Tofu:
- 1 14-oz. block extra-firm tofu, pressed and cubed
- 3 tbsp. cornstarch
- 1 tbsp. soy sauce
- 1 tbsp. sesame oil
- For the Sauce:
- Two cloves garlic, minced
- 2 tsp. cornstarch
- 2 tbsp. orange zest
- 3 tbsp. rice vinegar (or substitute with white vinegar)
- ½ cup of orange juice
- 1 tbsp. light soy sauce (you may substitute with tamari for a gluten-free recipe)
- 1 tbsp. Shaoxing wine
- 2 tbsp. sugar

- ¼ tsp. fine sea salt
- For the Stir fry:
- One head broccoli, chopped into bite-size pieces
- Two carrots, julienned

Directions:

To prepare the Tofu:

Mix the tofu with soy sauce and sesame oil to mix.

Sprinkle half of cornstarch over the tofu and mix. Repeat and make sure all the tofu is well coated.

Set the air fryer's temperature at 390 degrees Fahrenheit (unless the model doesn't require it).

Once hot, add the coated tofu to the air fryer basket and cook for 5 minutes.

When done, shake or stir the tofu.

Cook again for a further 5 minutes and set aside.

To stir fry:

Mix all the stir fry sauce Ingredients in a bowl.

Heat 1/4 cup of water in a large nonstick skillet over medium-high heat until the water boils.

Add the broccoli and carrots.

Cover then cook until the veggies are tender, about 1 to 2 minutes.

Let the water completely evaporate. Stir the sauce and then pour into the skillet.

Quickly stir for a few times until the sauce is thick and glossy.

Add the tofu and stir a few more times to mix well. Immediately transfer to a plate and serve to pipe hot over steamed noodles or rice.

Nutrition:

Total Calories: 298kcal

Carbohydrates: 32.4g

Protein: 16g

Fat: 12.6g

Potassium: 609mg

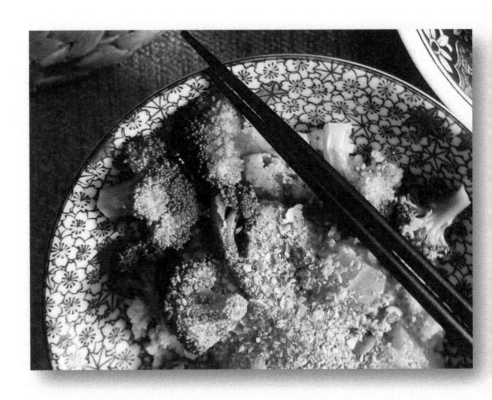

General Tso's Cauliflower Tofu

Skip the takeout! This version of General Tso's Cauliflower Tofu is super delicious and, best of all, healthy.

Preparation time: 15 minutes
Cooking time: 20 minutes
Servings: 2

Ingredients:

- For the primary chickpea binder:
- ½ cup chickpea flour
- ½ - 1 cup water or almond milk
- A pinch of salt.
- For the basic Panko breading:
- 1 cup Panko crumbs
- 1 - 2 tbsp. olive oil
- A pinch of salt.
- For the sauce:
- 3 tbsp. soy sauce or coconut aminos
- 2 tbsp. rice wine vinegar
- 2 tbsp. sherry
- 2 tsp. sesame oil
- 3 tbsp. agave nectar or sugar
- 1 tbsp. cornstarch
- ¼ cup veggie stock

- Dried chilli or chilli flakes, to taste
- Toasted sesame seeds
- Green onion, sliced thinly

Directions:

To prepare the chickpea binder:

In a prepared shallow dish, combine the chickpea flour and then slowly add water to the mix.

Continuously stir, removing any lumps using a fork until you reach the consistency of thin pancake batter.

Stir in a pinch of salt and set aside.

To prepare the panko breading:

In a shallow dish, combine the breadcrumbs and oil.

Use your hands or an oil brush to make sure the oil is evenly distributed, and add in a salt pinch.

To bread:

Prepare the vegetables or tofu into pieces.

Add the pieces to the chickpea binder and coat them thoroughly.

Transfer the pieces to the breading mixture, lightly press the breadcrumbs onto the parts, and then remove them to a tray.

To Air-Fry and Stir Fry:

Preheat and set the air fryer's temperature to 400 degrees Fahrenheit.

Cook the tofu or veggies for 10 - 20 minutes. Turn them as they cook to ensure they brown evenly. They should come out golden brown and crispy.

Combine all of the sauce Ingredients, right down to the chilli flake, in a bowl or measuring cup.

Stir until the cornstarch is well blended in.

Pour this mixture into a pan and on medium heat, and allow it to come to a simmer. Stir constantly.

If the sauce is thick and glossy, add the chilli.

Stir and allow to bubble for one more minute.

Turn off the heat and add the breaded and air fried pieces.

Mix well to combine.

Serve and garnished with sesame seeds and green onion.

Nutrition:

Energy (calories): 554 kcal

Protein: 14.87 g

Fat: 20.24 g

Carbohydrates: 77.46 g

Five Spice Tofu

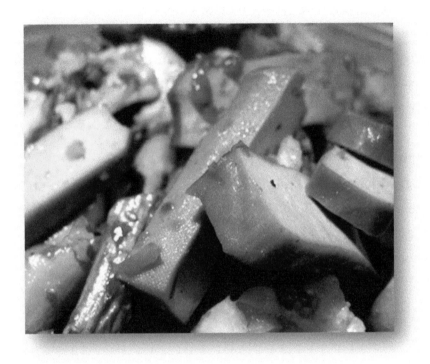

Preparation time: 10 minutes

Cooking time: 20 minutes

Servings: 4

Ingredients:

- 1 12-oz block extra-firm tofu
- 2 tbsp. oil
- For the Marinade:
- 1 tbsp. Chinese black vinegar + 1 tsp.
- 2 tsp. Chinese five-spice powder
- 2 tsp. garlic powder

- 1 tsp. Dark soy sauce
- ¼ cup maple syrup
- ½ tsp. salt or to taste

Directions:

Prepare the marinade Ingredients and mix in a large bowl.

Drain the tofu.

Wrap up the tofu in a clean kitchen paper towel and squeeze to remove excess water.

This will cause the tofu to crumble into chunks.

Add tofu to the marinade and mix until all the marinade is well absorbed.

Drizzle the oil over the tofu and mix. Prepare the air fryer basket by spraying it with cooking oil spray. This will ensure the tofu doesn't stick.

Transfer the tofu to the air fryer basket and cook at 400 degrees Fahrenheit for 20 minutes, shaking the basket halfway through cooking.

Serve piping hot.

Nutrition:

Energy (calories): 235 kcal

11%

Protein: 20.95 g

Fat: 11.62 g

Carbohydrates: 15.82 g